ALKALINE

DIET

Delicious Alkaline Diet Recipes For Weight Loss with Meal Plan to Cleanse Your Body

Martha Jensen

Published by David Kruse Publishing House

© Martha Jensen

All Rights Reserved

Alkaline Diet: Delicious Alkaline Diet Recipes For Weight Loss with Meal Plan to Cleanse Your Body

ISBN 978-1-989744-01-7

Legal & Disclaimer

The information contained in this book is not designed to replace or take the place of any form of medicine or professional medical advice. The information in this book has been provided for educational and entertainment purposes only.

The information contained in this book has been compiled from sources deemed reliable, and it is accurate to the best of the Author's knowledge; however, the Author cannot guarantee its accuracy and validity and cannot be held liable for any errors or omissions. Changes are periodically made to this book. You must consult your doctor or get professional medical advice before using any of the suggested remedies, techniques, or information in this book.

Upon using the information contained in this book, you agree to hold harmless the Author from and against any damages, costs, and expenses, including any legal fees potentially resulting from the application of any of the information provided by this guide. This disclaimer applies to any damages or injury caused by the use and application, whether directly or indirectly, of any advice or information presented, whether for breach of contract, tort, negligence, personal injury, criminal intent, or under any other cause of action.

You agree to accept all risks of using the information presented inside this book. You need to consult a professional medical practitioner in order to ensure you are both able and healthy enough to participate in this program.

TABLE OF CONTENTS

Part -1

Introduction

I want to thank you and congratulate you for downloading the book, "Alkaline Diet: A Guide For Improving Your Health Whilst Losing Weight and Balancing Your pH".

This book contains proven steps and strategies on how to maintain an Alkaline Diet.

Sometimes this may seem a bit too odd to be true. But as you keep your patience and read on through the following pages, you will soon start to discover that there are ways by which your body is affected by the amount of alkaline consumption that you are exposed to on a daily basis. This e-book will try to instruct you on how you can maintain the blood pH level in your body. When you change to an alkaline lifestyle, you can have the lean, trim body you've always wanted and experience a new level of wellness, energy and mental clarity, by utilizing this step-by-step guide.

Thanks again for downloading this book, I hope you enjoy it!

Chapter 1: What is the Alkaline Diet?

An alkaline diet is loosely based on the idea that the food you consume will change the acidity or alkalinity (which is the pH value) of your body. A healthy Alkaline Diet will always involve the ideal steadiness between acidifying and alkalizing foods.

Let us start with the facts first. Our body contains a vast number of systems that can counterweight and reduce excess acids, but however there is always a limit to how much acid our body can neutralize and even a limit to how much acid our body can cope with. The human body is capable of maintaining its daily pH balance provided the organs are working properly and a well-balanced alkaline diet is being consumed, while other acid-producing factors, such as tobacco use, are avoided.

First, let us try a little chemistry: A pH level can measure how acidic or alkaline something is. A pH of 0 is totally acidic, while a pH of 14 is completely alkaline. A pH of 7 is neutral. Those levels vary throughout your body. Your blood is slightly alkaline, while your stomach is very acidic, so it can break down food. And your urine changes and depending on what you eat–that's how your body keeps the level in your blood steady.

So what is the Alkaline food theory?

Alkaline food theory is the way of eating which recommends that the amounts of food that we eat in a daily diet should be based on our ability to adjust blood acidity or alkalinity.

The Alkaline diet is a comprehensive guide based on foods that are mainly alkaline forming. This can directly neutralize excess metabolic acids and make it possible to maintain a sustained health and immune capability.

Over time, as you follow the Alkaline Diet, it can help restore your digestive and immune system proficiency. You will become tolerant to, and can once again eat safely, the items to which your body had previously reacted.

Chapter 2: Why should you follow the Alkaline diet?

Can fat be an acid problem?

Recently I found out the cause of being overweight. Fat is caused by over-acidification.

What does that mean? The body will create fat cells to carry acids away from your vital organs which is actually a response from the body to an alarming over-acidic condition.

Why is being acidic harmful?

With an excess acid load, the delicate machinery of the human body does not work very well. This cellular machinery is delicately composed to work best within a slim, slightly alkaline range (pH: 7.35 - 7.55).

The proficiency of energy assembly in the cells is abridged with even slight excess of cell acid. This induces loss of flexibility and repair mechanisms, and you will become more susceptible to exhaustion, sickness, and discomfort, while your body tries to remove excess acid, critical minerals are lost as well.

These minerals will protect your kidneys, bladder, and ureter from acid impairment.

Following an Alkaline Diet will mean:

•choosing fresh, whole foods with certified organic and biodynamic being best choices. Examples will be provided on the next chapter.

•eating a wide variety of nutrients. Many people eat a limited variety of foods. A wider choice of foods is more interesting and will help to stimulate recovery. Whereas, the rotation of foods may be advised by your physician which will help. to relieve a weakened digestive system.

• Drinking lots of pure water which will rapidly excrete soluble wastes rather than allowing them to accumulate in your body.

- building your alkaline and mineral reserves. This will enhance the energy production, efficient protein production, and tissue repair.

Chapter 3: How to Maintain an Alkaline Body.

It is important for you to understand that an alkaline body will not mean the blood is more alkaline than normal. The pH of your blood is tightly regulated and will not differ except under risky, and often life-frightening, conditions.

Rather, an alkaline body will always refer to a body that requires little neutralization of acid in order to maintain blood at a constant pH. Urine is one of the ways by which the body rids itself of excess acids and for this reason naturopathic doctors will often measure the pH of an individual's urine in order to estimate how acid or alkaline their body is. A list of nourishments and their acid load are provided below. Many foods categorized as acidic, like nuts, whole grains, and lean protein sources, should be considered as part of a healthy diet. Some acidic foods can actually be a healthier choice than other more alkaline options. For example, whole wheat flour can be listed as highly acidic whereas refined flour is listed as mildly acidic.

Whole wheat flour however will always be a healthier choice despite the higher acidity because it is richer in vitamins, minerals, and fiber. Likewise, just because milk can be classified as neutral (neither acidic nor alkaline forming), does not mean it is appropriate for everyone. Try to use your best judgment so that you create a diet which balances healthy acidic foods with healthy basic foods to promote an alkaline body.

THE DIET:

•Follow the Alkaline Diet of mainly vegetables and fruits and try to avoid fried foods.

•Drink lots of water per day.

• Avoid alcohol, caffeine, soda, sugar, artificial sweeteners, additives, artificial colorings or seasonings and hydrogenated oil.

•Always minimize animal-based foods.

•Avoid pork, which can be difficult to digest and may create toxins in the body.

•Try to ignore the use of vegetable or corn oil for cooking as on heating them, may create toxins and irritation.

Chapter 4: The Meal Plans.

To make it easier for you to track down the Alkaline Diet targeted to particular health issues, I have created some meal plans for you. But first you will have to know the nitty-gritties. It is quite simple to develop nutritious, tasty meals encompassed mainly of alkalinizing foods. Below I have written down some examples of Alkaline meals. Breakfast can be a simple and stimulating meal, followed by a hearty lunch and dinner.

Ideally, you would benefit well to make lunch your main meal. This is mainly because your digestion will always be stronger during mid-day than at night. Below I will list various meal options that can serve as either lunch or dinner according to your personal preference.

Healthy Alkaline Menu Sample:

The following is a sample of a daily menu. It is not provided as a nutritional plan but simply as a reference of how alkaline and acidic foods can be combined to create an overall alkaline diet which will still provide adequate calories and proteins. Calorie needs vary from person to person so consult your doctor or a dietitian for a customized dietary plan that will meet your needs.

Breakfast

Buckwheat cereal with almond milk is quick and filling on a cold morning. Buckwheat groats, cracked or cream of buckwheat are available in most health food stores.

Steamed broccoli is an excellent choice for breakfast. Lightly steam broccoli for 5 minutes. You may add chopped onion and/or another green vegetable. Lightly stir in some Basic Salad Dressing and top with soaked almonds or hazelnuts. To soak nuts, place enough for the day in a container and cover with water. Place in the refrigerator overnight. Drain the next morning and enjoy. Rinse twice a day.

Basic Salad Dressing:

1/3 cup fresh lemon/lime juice

1 cup cold pressed extra virgin olive oil

½teaspoon ground oregano

½teaspoon ground cumin

½teaspoon garlic powder

½teaspoon Zip, by Spice Hunter (or a dash of cayenne pepper)

1-Tablespoon Bragg's Aminos

Lunch:

Salads are great for any meal. Keep spinach and leafy lettuces cleaned and place in a covered container, with a paper towel in the bottom and in the refrigerator. This way it feels like a salad is almost always ready to serve. Then build a salad with your choice of the following: fresh avocado, tomato, sprouts, green or purple onion, cucumber, celery, peppers, etc. Cut over the top some chunks of fresh firm tofu. Also add a few spoonful's of humus/salsa and then sprinkle with sunflower seeds or sliced almonds and then toss it with a basic salad dressing.

Dinner:

Preheat the oven to 200- C. Place a roasting tray to heat up the oven.

Cut the root vegetables into about 3cm sized dice and then coat with oil and season with salt and pepper. After that Put the vegetables onto the tray when it is hot and shake to dispense evenly. Roast them for around 40 mins.

Toast the coriander, fennel seeds and cumin in a dry frying pan for a few minutes and grind them to a rough powder and mix in the turmeric.

Put the chilli, ginger, garlic and onion in a blender and puree. Gently heat a splash of oil in a frying pan over a medium-low temperature and put in the spices. Fry for about a minute and add the paste. Stir for about 5 mins until the paste has soften and reduced in volume. Add more oil if needed.

Stir in the coconut milk and tomatoes. Add the cinnamon, simmer and stir constantly. Season to taste. Pour the sauce over the roasting vegetables.

Bake everything for about 25 mins, until the vegetables are tender and the sauce has thickened. Finish with fresh lime juice squeezed over it and garnish with fresh coriander leaves.

This curry dish is delicious by itself, but please feel free to serve it with brown basmati rice.

NOTE: MENU SUGGESTIONS ARE INTERCHANGABLE FOR ANY MEAL.

Chapter 5: The Liquid Diet.

LIQUIDS-ONLY NUTRIENT SUFFICIENCY PLAN:

The intestines of a typical person are always over-loaded, over-stressed, and over-exposed to various waste products. I would suggest that a major predisposition to chronic illness is created by the slow-transit mal-digestion, which has become an endemic in the Western industrialized countries during the last one or two generations. Rather, foods with restructured, processed, or immature fiber are kind of responsible for this. The way we move, and the kind of exercise we get, the way we breathe, and the way we adapt to stress in our lives also play significant roles. These are all habits that we learned.

With a bit of practice, life-sustaining habits can be learned. And these are the particular aspects of our lives that we can always influence by our own actions and attitudes.

The following are recommended:

•Miso Broth

Miso broth is a fully fermented product which is derived from soy and can be easily digested. The amino acids and other simple products are rarely a problem even for those with soy sensitivities.

•Juice from Watermelon

Watermelon juice is a surprisingly tasty drink made from blended ripe watermelon pieces (without seeds). A small amount of ginger tea or compatible liquid can be added to start the blending process. Other melons may also be used. This can be stored covered in the refrigerator for an entire day.

•Ginger Tea

Ginger tea is made from whole, fresh ginger root (increasingly available in more grocery produce areas). The best ginger root can be found in Hawaii. An easy way to make ginger tea is to freeze the fresh ginger, thaw until it is soft, slice and dice the juicy root, and boil in a warmed pot of hot water for ten minutes. Ginger tea is tasty at any temperature and can be stored refrigerated for several days in a very tightly sealed jar.

•Vegetable Juice

Vegetable juice can be an outstanding source of minerals, especially calcium, magnesium, potassium, and zinc, particularly if the vegetables are grown in rich, organic soil. Vegetables will always have a root system that will absorb and often concentrate whatever it is which is present in the soil, and any chemicals(if present) will be incorporated into the vegetable. Because of this absorption, it is important to obtain organic vegetables for juicing.

Carrot juice, which is the staple of vegetable juices can be drunk alone or can be combined with other vegetables.

Adding a half-inch of ginger root will increase the digestion of the juice and make it more alkaline. Try to change the proportions or dilute the juice to suit your palate. Let your sense of taste buds be your guide. The juice should taste hearty and delicious.

•Fruit Smoothies

Fruit smoothies are delightful when compatible with your"liquid days." Tree-ripened fruit, pitted and cut into wedges can be whipped into a tasty puree in your blender. However, the chosen fruits should be non-reactive with your immune system.

•Water

We all need it

•Herbal Teas

Herbal teas, alone or with a squeeze of citrus juice or a drop of raw honey, are welcome additions to this program.

[A reminder: This is not a fast. You should take in three or more quarts of fluid during the day and enough easily assimilated food building blocks to assuage hunger, enhance repair,

and rebuild.]

Chapter 6: Developing the Alkaline Diet

Guidelines for Developing Your Alkaline Diet:

If you are in an acid state, the first step is to eat more alkaline vegetables, fruits, spices, and lentils. Attempt for two cups of alkalinizing vegetables at both lunch and dinner. Trying to enjoy a breakfast of alkaline fruits or oatmeal while limiting high protein foods will also go a long way toward reducing your acidity. In addition, the following simple changes are especially helpful for quickly alkalinizing yourself:

•Drink the juice of one-half a lime, lemon, or a teaspoon of apple cider vinegar in 6-8 ounces of water a few times during the day. You may think this would make you more acidic. Instead, these substances metabolize to an alkaline residue due to the dicarboxylic acids that the body uses to make energy in a way that gives off an alkaline (bicarbonate) product.

•Add lentils, ginger, yams, and sweet potatoes to your diet on a regular basis as These foods will give you an alkaline boost.

•Make it a point to eat daily at least two cups of alkalinizing greens (kale, mustard and turnip greens, collards, or endive). Lettuce is fine to eat, but not in place of alkaline greens. Grated daikon radish is a wonderful alkalinizing condiment.

•Add miso and seaweed to soups and other dishes as both an amazing digestive aid and very alkaline.

•Eat more of the alkalinizing grains like oats, quinoa, and wild rice.

•Enjoy lots of amounts of fruits, especially watermelon.

•If you suffer from gas or weak digestion, try to eat cooked fruit and small amounts of fresh juices.

•Certain supplements like a fully buffered ascorbate (vitamin C), soluble (ionized) magnesium, and L-Glutamine [with Pyridoxal-alpha-ketoglutarate (PAK)] will also alkalinize you and should be used in doses as needed based on your metabolism. It has been found that an optimum dose of fully buffered ascorbate with a combination of calcium, magnesium, potassium, and zinc is a health-endorsing way to alkalinize, energize, and increase metabolism of toxins at the same time.

Be patient and determined. Remember, your pH indicates your reserve of alkaline minerals. An alkaline pH indicates good reserves of the enzyme-activating alkaline minerals. It can take time to build up these reserves.

It may take years to become depleted. Never be disheartened with a slow movement towards the ideal alkaline state—a first morning pH of 6.5 to 7.5.

For the body to effectively maintain its regular and slight alkaline balance, it will need a rich supply of alkalizing minerals. And, we need to eat food that doesn't overwhelm ourbody's natural ability to get rid of acid.

If you're recovering from an illness or chronic condition, the Alkaline Diet will infuse your body with much-needed nutrition to start the healing process, and it will remove the additional stresses that a bad diet can create.

For instance, according to the National Institutes of Health, diet is one of several factors that can contribute to kidney stone formation. Kidney stones can form when substances in the urine—such as calcium and phosphorus—become highly concentrated.

After the body uses what it needs from the food we eat for rejuvenation, the waste products in the bloodstream are carried to the kidneys and excreted as urine. It makes sense, then, that if our diet reduces these harmful substances and the kidneys don't have to work as hard to stabilizethe acid-alkaline level in your body, they'll be able to evadekidney stones. Also, if your thyroid isn't busy handling stress hormones released because of the food you eat, it will be better able to function. Our thyroids regulate many of the hormones in the body, including those that affect our metabolism. In this way, one can achieve and sustain a healthy immune system and overall health.

Conclusion

Thank you again for downloading this book!

I hope this book was able to help you to follow the Alkaline Diet.

The next step is to take action on everything that you've learnt in this book.

Thank you and good luck!

Part – 2

Introduction

Sadly enough, we live in an age where people feel less and less healthy as the days go by. The truth is that there are many contributing factors to the generally unhealthy state of most of the people out there, but that our alimentation is one of the primary ones.

What do we do?

We wake up, jump in our cars or take a subway, go to work or school, come back home, open the TV or the computer, waste our times in front of it and then go to sleep so that the next day follows the same pattern. And in between all these "activities", all we do is eat badly: no breakfast other than one cup of coffee, a lunch that is either completely unhealthy or almost inexistent and a copious dinner usually comprised out of fast-food or pre-processed meals. No wonder our bodies are weakening!

What should we do?

You must have heard this before a thousand times at least, but it is the actual truth: you have to exercise and you have to eat healthier. This is the only way in which you can restore your body's health condition.

However, things are much trickier than they may seem to anyone who has not tried this before. In between fad diets promising to help you lose 20 pounds in 5 days and nutritionists that have gained this title overnight, it is difficult to actually select the information that is worthy of your attention. Even more than that, not only much of what is out there on the topic of nutrition is pure make-believe and incorrect, but some of the so-called "diets" may actually be harmful for your body instead of helping it heal itself.

So, what is there to do?

The alkaline diet comes up with a solution that is based on actual studies made in the field of nutrition and which will not promise you to simply help you "lose weight", but to actually restore your health to its optimum level.

Do not feel tempted to believe that this will be easy and that you will be able to switch to the alkaline diet the same way as you switch your computer on or off. However, do believe in the power this diet has when it comes to changing your life. Every single part of your body will benefit out of it and your mental state will improve as a consequence too.

Will it be difficult?

Maybe, depending on how you feed yourself right now. But the results will definitely pay off your effort. You will feel better from so many points of view that you will start asking yourself why you haven't done this sooner. Step by step, your old diet will become just a faded memory and once you see the benefits of the alkaline diet you will not want to go back to your old eating habits any longer simply because you will see how much your state will improve.

This book aims at providing you with the basic and useful information you need in order to get yourself going on the alkaline diet. While there will be plenty of other sources of information on this topic as well, this book is meant for those of you who have never heard of the alkaline diet before and who would like to give it a try.

Do not give up! Health is just one step away and all you have to do is reach out and grab it by the hand!

Chapter 1: The Basics

For someone who has never heard of the alkaline diet, even the basics of this lifestyle will sound either odd or just confusing. However, do not fear, because things are much easier to understand than it may seem at first. The alkaline diet can be explained simply so that you can understand what it is that you should actually do about it.

Basically, the alkaline diet is a nutrition plan which attempts at eliminating (as much as possible) products that create acid in the blood. This diet focuses on eating as many fruits, vegetables, legumes and nuts as possible, while at the same time it focuses on trying to avoid meat, poultry, dairy and grains.

To understand why you should avoid these products, you should first and foremost think of what our human ancestors ate. Grains and products made out of grains started to be familiar to humans only during the stone age, dairy products started to be familiar only when humans started to settle down and domesticate cattle, salt and sugar started to be consumed on large scales when the technology behind extracting these seasonings started to develop more (especially during the industrial age in the case of sugar) and meat and poultry may have been eaten, but in much smaller quantities than they are today simply because birds and livestock had not been domesticated yet.

On the large scale of things, all these foods are very recent for our bodies and this is precisely why they have not adjusted to the new "regimen" yet. Yes, it may seem silly that the human body has not adapted to digesting and transforming into energy so many foods in thousands of years, but the truth is that the evolutionary process is a lengthy one and that all these thousands of years feel like the split of a second for the evolution of all species.

Enough with the history lesson though. To understand how the alkaline diet works in even more depth, you will have to go back to your basic Chemistry lessons for a bit (to that lesson which taught you about pH). In Chemistry, alkaline solutions are considered to be the opposite of the acidic ones. Whenever the alkalinity of a solution is higher, the acidity is likely to be low and the other way around. While in Chemistry maintaining the balance between the two of them may not be important (and sometimes lack of balance may even be artificially created), in Biology/Anatomy this has started to be an issue more and more specialists are looking into.

The relationship between alkalinity/acidity and what our human ancestors ate should not be difficult to understand. The human body is not adjusted to high levels of acidity and most of the foods eaten by the vast majority of people out there transform themselves into acid when they are de-composed by the human digestive system. At the same time, people eat less and less fruits, vegetables and other alkaline-based products, which consequently leads to a rise in the level of acidity (which, as you will later on see, can affect every part of your body and it can lead to the development of various medical conditions as well).

You will also want to know the fact that the alkaline diet went through 2 main phases, each with its own theory on why the human body needs a perfect balance between alkaline substances and acidic ones.

The traditional theory sustains the idea that foods such as meat, poultry, eggs, milk, cheese, fish and grains lead to a high acidity in the body, while foods such as vegetables and fruits (except for prunes, cranberries and plums) lead to a higher alkalinity. However, the traditional view on this matter is also based on the idea that the body maintains its natural pH with a relatively small amount of effort.

The more modern theory advances the traditional one and sustains the idea that high acidity can lead to the development of osteoporosis. The "mechanism" behind this idea is based on the fact that whenever the body feels that the intake in acidic-rich foods is too high, it will try to buffer this with the help of one of its 3 main buffer systems: the protein one, the carbon acid – bicarbonate one and the phosphate one. One of these 3 buffer systems also involves breaking down the bones, which consequently leads to osteoporosis.

This theory has been advanced in many expert circles and it has started to be widely acknowledged. Even more, certain health institutions recommend a large intake of fruits and vegetables precisely due to their alkaline richness and due to the fact that this is supposed to balance out the acidity in the body (and thus protect it from the development of osteoporosis).

Another thing you will have to understand is related to the fact that you should *not* believe that an extremely high level of alkalinity is actually healthy. In fact, the alkaline diet is not seeking to increase the alkalinity of your body fluids, but to bring balance in your body when it comes to its pH.

Since blood plasma is slightly alkaline, acidity in blood is not healthy. Even more, you should bear in mind the fact that the natural and optimal pH of your body's fluids is of something in between 7.35 and 7.45 and that the body works hard to maintain it this way. If the pH drops under these levels, the body develops a condition known as acidosis. Likewise, if the pH rises above these levels, the condition the body develops will be called alkalosis. If the pH drops below 7.0 or rises above 7.8, death can occur.

Chapter 2: How to Tell If Your Body is

Acidic

If this entire relationship between alkalinity and acidity in your body is new to you, then you may wonder on how you can determine if your body is threatened by its own acidity. If you want to find this out, then follow the next tips and you will be able to tell if your body is acidic or not:

Frequent pain that occurs without an apparent reason can be a sign of acidity in the body.

Frequent colds or catching the flu too often can also be a sign of too much acid in the body.

Heartburn (burning sensation right between your heart and your stomach) is another sign of poor digestion (and thus of a potentially acidic body).

Kidney stones are also a sign in very many cases.

Receding gums are very frequently a sign of too much acid in the body as well.

To determine exactly whether or not your body is acidic, there are two types of tests you can take:

· The saliva test. This test will require you to buy special pH determining bands from your local pharmacy. Test your saliva the very first thing in the morning. At this time of the day, your pH should be of around 6.8 to 7.2 but it can very often remain at 6.8 or even a bit lower than that. Further on, test your saliva immediately after a meal as well (leave 5 minutes in between the meal and the test though). At this point, the pH should be between 6.8 and 8.4. Then, test your saliva after 2 more hours. At this point, the pH should be between 6.8 and 7.2 If you consistently see that the pH levels are very low, then it may mean that your body does not have enough alkaline nutrients in it to counter-balance the acidity.

· The urine test. You can use the same type of test strips as for the saliva test as well. Test your urine first thing in the morning and then another time when you have to urinate the second time in the day. Calculate the average between the two results. A healthy body pH should be around 6.8 and 7.2.

In both of these cases, make sure that you test yourself over a period of time (one week at least), so that you can get a realistic view on how healthy your body is (or not).

Chapter 3: Why Choose the Alkaline Diet?

Now that you understand the basics behind the alkaline diet, you may wonder why exactly you should choose it over all the other diets out there. Even more, you may wonder why exactly it is that you should change your diet. Of course, you may understand the fact that a high level of acidity or an imbalance in your body will not be the healthiest thing for it, but what exactly are the effects of the alkaline diet? How will it change your life and why have other people chosen it?

There are many benefits that result from following the alkaline diet. Here are some of the most commonly reported ones (by those who have already went on the diet):

Your immunity will be improved and even the banal cold will stay farther from your body.

Your energy levels will increase. Even if you do not necessarily take into consideration the basic idea behind the alkaline diet, eating many fruits and vegetables will actually increase the level of your energy.

If you suffer from chronic pain of any kind (including the chronic fatigue syndrome for example), you will start feeling much better because your health state will ameliorate considerably.

Your body will assimilate nutrients much better (which will consequently make you feel much better as well).

The alkaline diet can help you detoxify your body of all those harmful elements that "got stuck" in it.

Your mental state will improve as well and it has been reported that those on the alkaline show more mental acuity and mental alertness.

Studies show that an alkaline-based diet can also reduce candida as well.

You will sleep much better because your body will come back to its natural way of functioning.

Your skin will look more youthful and more elastic (and all through natural and healthy nutrition!).

You will be able to control your blood sugars better – definitely a great health benefit.

High acidity can lead to acidic reflux, to gastrointestinal pain, to ulcer and to bowel health issues. Going on the alkaline diet can help you ameliorate these conditions as well.

If you suffer from high blood pressure, there is a very high chance that the condition will be improved as well.

It can reduce osteoporosis and it can help ameliorating arthritic pain as well.

The cholesterol levels will also be reduced, which will consequently help your circulatory system function better and it will reduce the chance that you develop Diabetes.

Many people who suffer from cancer have reported that their health condition got better after switching to the alkaline diet.

You can lose weight by going on the alkaline diet. Certain studies show that weight gain and being overweight may actually be related to the acidity level in your body's fluids.

All in all, the alkaline diet can change your life to the better. Months from starting the diet in the first place, you will feel like the older and energy-lacking you is a very bad dream and that you were always meant to be this way: healthy, full of energy and liveliness. And the truth is that we are all created to function this way – it's just that bad nutrition brings us down.

The following chapters will describe the way in which the alkaline diet can influence some of the medical conditions out there and how they are related to high levels of acids in the body fluids. Knowing all these things is very important because it will motivate you to actually stick to this diet (even if you do not necessarily suffer from any of those medical conditions). Even more, it will help you understand your body better and it will help you understand that giving it what it truly needs (real food) will benefit you from all points of view.

Chapter 4: Acidity Your Body's Number

One Enemy

In the previous chapters it has been pointed out the fact that acidity can harm your body. Even more than that, several of the well-known benefits of the alkaline diet have also been pointed out.

This chapter is dedicated to understanding how acidity can interact with your bones, with your circulatory system and with various other parts of your body that will simply stop functioning in the normal parameters once acidity is installed in the body.

Bones

It has been mentioned that under certain circumstances, the human body reacts to the acidic waste gathered in it by breaking down the bones. While it may not actually "break" the bones, acidity leads to something that is similar to it. Basically, when the body senses that the blood alkalinity is affected by the acidic waste, it will try to protect itself by binding the acids with calcium (one of the alkaline nutrients that naturally occur in the human body). This will lead to the formation of calcium sediments that will be deposited around the bone structure and which will lead to pain (such as arthritis) and to other symptoms as soon as the human in whose body this happened starts to age.

Cardiovascular System

To understand the relationship between acidic waste and the cardiovascular system, think of vandals who want to escape a closed yard. Instead of waiting for someone to open the gate for them, they will start attacking the wall, with the hope of breaking it sooner or later. This works the same with acids in blood as well. When there is too much acid in one's blood and the body cannot make enough calcium deposits, the acids will attack the arteries. To repair this damage, the body will try to "cover up" the "wounds" with whatever it finds in near vicinity: triglycerides, cholesterol, calcium and so on. This is how arteries thicken up eventually and how many people get to suffer from circulatory diseases that can require life-long treatment, surgery and that can even lead to death.

Immunity

Acid waste can also play "tricks" on the immune system as well. Basically, when a certain type of food is not suitable for a particular body, the immune system will try to produce histamines and to lead certain enzymes to create slips through the intestines. Once the bad foods slip through, the immune system is ready to "annihilate" them. However, this comes with a huge price: the immune system turns against the body and it starts attacking its protoplasm. There are numerous auto-immune diseases that can be caused by the same pattern: Cron's disease, Celiac disease, Lupus, rheumatoid arthritis (yes, this is an auto-immune disease) and many other diseases which are fully recognizes as stand-alone medical conditions.

Cancer

Probably one of modern day's most feared and most mysterious disease at the same time, cancer has yet to find its cure. While it may not be known exactly how cancerous cells develop in the human body, one thing is for sure: cancer does kill and in most of the cases it is discovered late enough as to not even allow the patient to obtain some form of treatment.

Those who sustain the alkaline diet have come up with a viable theory on how cancerous cells develop. Basically, when there is too much acid waste in the body and when it is located near certain organs (liver, kidney and so on), it will deposit on the caterpillars that are supposed to fuel those organs with the necessary nutrients. When the cells in the organs are not properly fed with nutrients and when there is little oxygen for them, they have two options: die or adapt. However, adaptation is not a good thing under these circumstances because the cells adapt to an environment which lacks oxygen – which consequently leads them to becoming malignant.

Of course, the development of cancer may be more complex than even the most important researchers in the world can understand at the moment. However, more and more research reveals that a diet low in acids can definitely slow down the cancerous cells precisely because it deprives them of the environment for which they have adapted themselves.

There are many diseases and medical conditions that can be affected by the acid waste in the body. The ones described here are the most important ones, but the truth is that there are scientists who suggest that almost every single health condition in the human body may be related to acidic waste first and foremost. If this idea would manage to reach more people, more of them would start feeling better about whatever condition it is that they suffer from.

Excessive Weight

Being overweight is not just about appearance and it should never be considered a matter of fashion only. Being overweight is one of the biggest threats brought to the human body and the harsh truth is that an alarming people in the Western countries (United States of America, United Kingdom and so on) suffer from obesity and even from morbid obesity.

So much extra-weight can put your life on hold. It can make you feel much less energetic, it can make you feel like lacking self-confidence and it can make you feel depressed and anxious. Even more than that, being overweight is very frequently related to heart diseases, to Diabetes and to numerous other medical conditions that can actually threat your life.

The alkaline diet can help you lose those extra-pounds. Although you should not primarily direct your focus on weight loss when it comes to this diet, losing weight will come as a natural consequence of eating healthier and of providing your body with what it truly needs. Restrictive calorie diets and "miracle" pills will do nothing good for your body. They can harm it, they can weaken it and in most of the cases they will lead to the famous yo-yo effect (putting back the weight you loss even faster than before). However, the alkaline diet is a balanced diet that will provide you with all the nutrients necessary for living and it will restore your body to its original form (on the inside and on the outside as well).

Chapter 5: Mental Status and Acidity

It may seem odd to some, but acidity has also been connected with various mental disorders and diseases. The fact that nutrition can affect one's mental status should not be a surprise though and it should be widely acknowledged by everybody out there.

There are particular disorders/diseases that get associated with acidity more often than others. Although a high level of acidity does not necessarily mean that you will automatically develop any of these conditions, it is good to be cautious and to change something in your life now, before it is too late. Here are some of the most common mental and neurological disorders associated with high acidity in the body:

Depression is considered to be the disease of the century and although it is not considered to be an actual disease any longer (but a disorder), the harsh truth is that it can affect everyone regardless of age, sex, nationality, location, financial status and so on.

Depression is a very serious issue and it can endanger one's life when it reaches a critical stage. More recently, even children have been discovered to suffer from depression and the world is already familiar with too many cases of children committing suicide.

Alzheimer's disease is another very much feared cognitive disease that affects short-term memory to the point where the patient forgets almost everything in his/her life.

Modern medicine associates Alzheimer's with certain beta-amyloid plaques that form in between the neurons' membranes. These proteins that stock up in the brain are somewhat similar to the way in which the arteries become thicker (as described in the previous chapter), especially when it comes to their susceptibility to high acidity. Thus, an important number of the researchers in this field nowadays associate high acidity to Alzheimer's and they believe that a nutrition rich in alkaline products and poor in acidic ones can prevent the onset of this disease and that it can even slow it down and ameliorate it in those cases which are not very severe.

Epilepsy is one of the most mysterious and yet feared mental disorders out there. Nobody has been able to come up with a theory to be unanimously accepted when it comes to the way in which epilepsy develops.

All specialists know is related to the fact that people who suffer from epilepsy show a high level of electricity in their brains (even when they are not undergoing a seizure). Some have suggested that the high level of electricity in the brain is associated with the fact that the neurons need to work much faster and they thus generate more electricity than normally. Also, these people usually suggest the fact that this unusual brain activity may as well be related in one way or another to high acidic levels of the body and that nutrition should be taken into consideration when managing epilepsy.

Do bear in mind the fact that these are just some of the mental and neurological disorders that have started to be associated with a high level of acidity in the body. Although research is still being made on this topic, the truth is that these theories are more viable than anything that has been developed up to the moment on these topics and that they may actually function.

Chapter 6: It Is Time to Detox Your Body

If your dietary habits have not been the best ones up to the moment, there is a high chance that you will discover that your body contains too much acidic waste. The main idea is that you should not despair, because these things can be fixed in time.

Of course, you will have to dedicate yourself to this cause. You will have to make sure to eat as healthy as humanly possible. You will have to make sure to remove those bad foods from your diet. You will have to make sure to stay strong even when you are craving for yet another fast food menu and another large soda.

Before even proceeding with explaining what it is that you should eat (and maybe even more importantly, *why* it is that you should eat that), you will first and foremost have to understand one simple fact: it is that you should eat that), you will first and foremost have to understand one simple fact: *improving your state of health lies in your power*. It will not be easy, but the results will be amazing. There will be times when you may want to jump back into your old lifestyle as well, but do remember that your bad habits brought you where you are today. Regardless of the reason behind this choice, that of following the alkaline diet, you should always make sure that you wake up every day with one main goal in mind: health. Your body needs real food that it can digest properly and even if you may not have noticed this until now, your body is also giving you a lot of signs on what it is that you should do. You need to listen to your inner calling because your body really knows what is best for its own good state and it will trigger you as soon as you eat something bad.

So, what is it that you should eat, what is it that you should not eat and why are certain foods so good or so bad for your health? Read on and find out the most important things you should keep in mind regarding your nutrition from now on.

Fruits and Vegetables

While nobody says that you should go full vegan (or at least not from the start, since a lot of people out there naturally lean towards vegan diets once they get accustomed with their new lifestyle), you should also know the fact that fruits and vegetables are absolutely essential for a good nutrition. Why is that?

Fruits and vegetables are the primary source of quality alkaline nutrients (calcium, magnesium, potassium, and so on). They fill you up, they are incredibly varied and tasty, they can be cooked in thousands of ways, they can make for a great snack, for a great smoothie, for a great dinner and for a great life in general.

Fruits and vegetables energize you and one of the reasons you may be feeling low energy at the moment may be related precisely to the fact that, like most of the people in the Western countries, you eat less and less fruits and vegetables as days go by. And no, store-bought juice does not classify as "fruit" or "vegetable" because it is filled with sugars and additives that simply make your body's condition worse (instead of improving it).

Ideally, you should eat at least 2-3 portions of fruits every day and 7-8 portions of vegetables every day as well. This may seem like a lot, but if you take a look at the variety of recipes that can be cooked with vegetables, you will realize that taking in so much of them is actually doable. As for fruits, it may be advisable to keep the number of portions lower because although fruits are incredibly delicious and healthy, they still contain fructose, which is a type of sugar. Especially for those of you suffering from Diabetes, a high intake of fructose is to be avoided. Do check with your doctor on this matter since he/she will be able to tell you more about how many fruits you are actually allowed to eat in one day.

Even more than that, there is yet another benefit to eating as many fruits and veggies as possible: they contain antioxidants that stop premature aging, they contain ingredients that are considered to be anti-inflammatory and they even contain ingredients that are considered to be able to fight cancer.

Your circulatory system will definitely thank you for having made the choice of incorporating more fruits and vegetables into your diet precisely because, as also mentioned before, a body that contains acidic waste will also be susceptible to high levels of cholesterol, triglycerides and, eventually, it can be susceptible to develop thick arteries.

The best way in which you can reap all the benefits fruits and vegetables can offer you with is to make sure that you only eat organic products. Fruits and vegetables that have been previously treated with various pesticides and solutions to boost their growth are unhealthy and they do not even taste as good as real food does.

Do not be afraid of trying out new recipes and of eating as many vegetables as possible. Even if you do have to lose weight, eating two pounds of vegetables (which is a lot indeed) will not even get close to the minimum amount of calories your body needs in order to sustain itself through one day. So, if you are trying to lose weight, you should definitely befriend veggies because they can be allies impossible to actually equal.

Fats

It may be surprising for you to read this, but the truth is that fat is not as bad as it was previously suggested in various medical researchers. Up until not very long ago, most of the medical professionals agreed upon the fact that fat should be avoided as much as possible because they associated it with colon and rectal cancer.

However, although many people still suggest that a low fat and high fiber diet is the suitable one for anyone who wants to avoid these two types of cancer, the situation may look completely different under the light of the more recent research made on this issue.

Basically, studies show that people who follow a low fat and high fiber diet are not more or less prone to develop colon cancer than those who eat more fat. Of course, this does not mean that you should indulge in all the fatty products out there, but it means that you are allowed to find the perfect balance for your body when it comes to the fat intake.

Even more than that, it has been shown that fiber cannot be assimilated into the body if there is no fat in the colon to help disintegrate it. Thus, it is not only allowed that you consume at least a small amount of fats and/or oils, but it is also advisable to do so.

And if you want to be even more amazed, you should know the fact that fats are absolutely essential for the well-being of your entire organism and not just when it comes to dissolving soluble fiber into the colon. Fat is crucial in producing cellular energy, in making the bile function well and in producing the right types of hormones. Furthermore, fat is the element which allows your body to digest proteins coming from meat and it is also an important element in maintaining your immune system in order.

Another reason for which many of the medical specialists out there advise against consuming products that contain fats is related to the fact that it was believed that clogged arteries are a direct result of consuming too much fat. However, it was more recently discovered that fat only "clings" to the arteries because they are already damaged (as also explained previously in the book).

So, what kinds of fats should you eat?

You should make sure that your fat intake is not too small because it can harm your body and it will not help it either. Take your fats from good sources, such as olive oil, salmon, tuna, red meat (but only if you know your body digests it well), nuts and from all those foods that are generally considered to contain the so-called "good fats". These fats will help your body function properly and they will also fuel your mind for better results as well.

However, do bear in mind the fact that there are two main types of bodies out there and that they will determine what kind of sources you should use for your fat intake. For instance, those of you who have a meat-eating metabolism (and can digest meat properly) will find that eating meat 4-5 times every week and allowing it to have a moderate amount of fat on it will work better. At the same time, those of you who have a grain-eating metabolism will find that fish is better when it comes to the fatty intake.

Fiber

While explaining fats and their role for the human body, it was mentioned that advising people to eat a high fiber and low fat diet may not be as healthy as some believe. However, do bear in mind that this should not mean that you eliminate all types of fiber from your life and that you should acknowledge the importance of fiber as well.

Basically, fiber is good for your body because it can help you manage certain medical conditions much better than normally. It has been shown that fiber is very important when it comes to preventing degenerative diseases and it has also been shown that fiber is a good helper for those who suffer from type II Diabetes (as those who consumed more fiber had a lower level of cholesterol and triglycerides in their bodies and they also showed closer to normal blood sugar levels as well).

Do bear in mind the fact that you should take your fiber from healthy sources, such as apples, carrots and foods that are rich in this element because simply eating bread may cause you to feel bad (especially if you are gluten-sensitive as well).

Sugars

It can be very hard to give up on sugar, especially if you have a sweet tooth and if you like eating cakes, cookies and other products that are normally very rich in sugar. While nobody says that you should live a "sour" life, you should also know the fact that refined sugars are truly harmful for your body from many points of view.

Excessively eating sugar can lead to the development of Diabetes. Even more than that, sugars are considered to be highly acidic as well, which adds up to their disadvantages.

Another health condition with which sugars are very frequently associated is called Candida Albicans. This infection can lead to many other diseases which can actually affect the overall health status of your body in incredibly harmful ways. Removing sugars from your diet can help you control this infection and restore your health.

Do bear in mind the fact that removing sugars from your life does not only include not eating sweets any longer. In fact, foods such as pasta and rice are considered to be very high in sugar levels and so are soft drinks, alcoholic drinks and many other products out there. You may be surprised by the fact that in most of the cases even the supermarket mustard and ketchup are full of sugars (not to mention fast food products, where even salad is "bathed" in sugar as well).

If you cannot give up on the sweet taste (and this would be perfectly normal), then you should know the fact that there are some very good replacements out there that will satisfy your sweet tooth. You can use them with your coffee or tea and you can also add them to your favorite homemade cakes that usually require sugar. Raw honey and stevia are among the most commonly used sugar-like ingredients out there and the truth is that they are natural, healthy and delicious at the same time – so they will make your path to health easier from this point of view at least.

Also, do try to avoid artificial sweeteners at all costs because all they do is bring additives and chemicals into your body and that is the last thing you want if you are on your path to becoming healthier. As for pasta and rice, you should substitute them with their wholegrain and brown alternatives because they will maintain the taste and the texture of the pasta while avoiding their disadvantages.

If you are in the mood to crunch on something in front of a movie, then it will be healthier for you if you chose nuts, seeds, baked apples and other similar things instead of cookies.

Also, avoid soft drinks at all costs because they are incredibly acidic and they will provide your body with absolutely no nutrients at all. They can ruin your stomach, they can ruin your energy levels (although they will not initially appear to do so), they can make you gain weight, develop various diseases and, in general, they are considered to be nothing but harmful for the human body.

Proteins

Although the alkaline diet advocates for eating as many fruits and vegetables as possible, this does not mean that you should give up on proteins. Do understand the fact that proteins may not always come from animal sources and that there are certain vegetables out there that are considered to have a high percentage of protein as well. Even more, if you do not want to (or cannot) give up on meat and poultry, you should not try to eliminate it completely from your life, but you should try to limit it to what your body truly needs.

The harsh truth is that most of the people who live in Western countries consume much more proteins than their bodies really need, which consequently leads to lack of balance in their bodies. What the average man or woman needs is no more than 0.8 mg protein for every pound they weigh. The average portion is somewhere around the size of your palm without fingers (for pork and generally fattier meat) and around the size of your palm with fingers (for fish and poultry that does not contain a lot of fat).

The best type of meat to eat is the white one (poultry, chicken, fish) and the worst one is, as you may expect, pork. This type of meat is too high in cholesterol and it has been linked with various medical conditions out there. Even more than that, it can be infested and it will be very difficult to digest too. Generally speaking, poultry is easier to digest and it is of the highest quality when it has been organically fed because this way you make sure that the animal was not fed with various additives that increase its weight in an unnatural way.

If you want to try to give up on meat completely, then you should also get familiar with those foods that are not of animal origins and which are also extremely rich in protein. Among these vegetables, you will find mushrooms, pea proteins, spirulina proteins, bananas and many, many other products out there. However, if you do stick to eating dairy products, always keep in mind that you should keep your cheese eating under control because in most of the cases cheese is too acidic for a healthy diet.

Debatable Foods

There are certain groups of foods that are highly debated among the nutritionist circles out there. These foods are considered to be either bad or good for the body and although the "fight" has not settled yet, there are certain things you should keep in mind about these foods.

Acid-tasting (or sour-tasting) foods, such as lemons and citric fruits in general, are acidic as well. However, you should know that a large part of those who have studies the alkaline diet believe that these fruits are actually alkaline.

Another group of foods that is much debated out there is that which contains spinach, bananas, artichokes, bananas, asparagus and so on. On the one hand, certain specialists believe that these foods should be avoided because they produce acid in the body. However, on the other hand there are specialists who believe that they should recommend these foods because they leave behind more alkaline substances in the body than they leave acidic ones.

Processed Food

As you have noticed up to the moment, nothing is fully prohibited in the alkaline diet and the key lies in finding the balance between the alkaline food intake and the acidic one. However, if there is one thing that should be 100% forbidden for anyone out there (outside of soda), that would be processed foods.

The harm these foods can bring into your body is difficult to imagine, but sadly this is how most of the people in the West eat. From frozen and pre-made products to the gummy bears we give our children, all of these processed foods contain a high dose of additives that ruin the natural balance of the body and bring it to the point of collapse.

You should avoid processed food at all times because it can have terrible effects on your health. Some people even associate them with several forms of cancer, but in addition to that you will suffer digestive issues, you will gain weight and you will feel less energetic, which are some of the main symptoms an acidic body shows.

Going alkaline will most likely help you and your body get rid of any toxicity. Even if giving up on your current lifestyle will seem very hard to do, the truth is that it is something you just have to do if you don't want to come back to the alkaline diet when your physical state has already degraded too much.

So, now that you know what you should eat and what you should not eat, you can easily build meal plans that will work into your new lifestyle. It may be confusing at first, but if you keep in mind the basics you will always find a reason. To help you, here is a list of some of the most alkaline-rich foods out there:

Honey (preferably raw because it is healthier)

Broccoli (this is great because you can cook it in many, many ways and you can even make it fun and delicious enough for your kids to like it as well).

Watermelon (this is one of the greatest desserts to replace your usual cupcakes or cookies and it will be more than affordable in the summer; even more, it is very healthy for the kidneys and it helps purifying them properly).

Green beans (you can cook them in various ways as well, from salad to actual slow cooker)

Hazelnuts (and nuts in general as well).

Tomatoes (you can easily incorporate them into your diet because they are present in many recipes and they can be eaten as such and in salads as well).

Cauliflower (works great with a bit of cheese on top and cooked into the oven with various spices).

Cucumber (this is again a very easy to incorporate food for those who are just starting out with the alkaline diet).

Kale (works great in salads, but you can also make kale chips by cooking the leaves into the oven until they become crisp – a great alternative to packaged potato chips).

Potatoes (it may be better to choose sweet potatoes instead of normal potatoes, especially if you are allergic to gluten which is found in high quantities in normal potatoes).

Onions (you may not eat them as such but again, they are part of many recipes out there and they can add savor and taste to almost anything).

Peppers (great in salads and they work great with different types of stuffing as well).

Apple (the old saying "one apple a day keeps the doctor away makes much more sense now, doesn't it?).

Berries (they work great with yogurt in the morning, but if you are also on a dairy-free diet, you can replace the yogurt with something else, you can add the berries to your oatmeal or you can simply eat them as such since they are delicious and refreshing in the morning).

Peaches (again, they make for a great snack for someone with a sweet tooth, especially when they are ripe and red-colored).

Lemons (as mentioned, they are alkaline, not acidic).

Tofu cheese (a great replacement for the other types of cheese that tend to be very high in acids).

Almonds (great to snack on or to add to your morning cereal for example).

Cinnamon (you will love this on your baked apples because it adds that special Christmas-like flavor of your average apple pie without also adding the sugars, the carbs and the extra-calories).

Curry (you can make hundreds and hundreds of recipes based on curry and Indians know this very well, as they tend to use this spice on the vast majority of their traditional foods).

Mustard (if you do buy it though, always make sure that it does not contain extra-sugar and that it is as natural as possible).

Sea salt (this is a great friend for those with hypertension and for those with kidney issues as well).

Ginger (you can make a great natural beverage out of it and as long as you do not add extra sugar, it can definitely replace your soda; also, it is widely used in various recipes out there too).

Chapter 7: The Perfect Alkaline Diet

Recipes

The wrong way to start any diet is by thinking that the things you will be eating from now on will be less tasty in any way than the things you used to eat up until the moment. This is a very bad attitude and it can completely ruin everything as it will persist "living" in the back of your head and it will constantly make you think of the fact that what you are eating does not actually have a good taste.

With the alkaline diet, you will not have anything to complain about when it comes to the taste of your foods. Since only soda and processed foods are completely forbidden, you are allowed to eat almost anything you may wish for and that is definitely an advantage over the rest of the diets that tend to be much more restrictive than this.

Even more, alkaline diet recipes are absolutely delicious and they will be quite easy to prepare as well. To give you an idea of the wide variety of things you can cook on this diet, just read on. You will definitely find the following recipes to be attractive for you!

Asian Soup

Asian food can be very tasty even without the excessive soy sauce and without the excessive oil and grease. There are many recipes out there that are much healthier and some of them are even very much alkaline-friendly as well. This soup is one of them. Easy to make and very good, this Asian soup will be something you will want to try again and again.

To make it, you will need the following ingredients: 4 cups water (it is preferable that it is filtered), 3 tablespoons braggs liquid aminos, 1 teaspoon grated ginger, 1 clove grated garlic, 1/8 teaspoon sea salt, 1 ½ cups shelled edamame beans, 3 cups chopped baby bok choy (use the stems and the greens as well), 80 oz udon noodles and green onions (these ones are optional).

Start by bringing together the water, the briggs, the ginger, the garlic, the salt and the edmame beans to medium heat. Meanwhile, cook the noodles as it is described on the package. Bring the bok choy to the broth for 1 minute and then split the vegetables, the broth and the noodles into equal parts and serve hot.

Grapefruit Salad

As mentioned previously in this book, citric fruits are very much welcomed into the alkaline diet. This salad will combine elements that may be surprising for some of you, but in the end you will get used to it and you will even learn to love it.

To make this particular type of grapefruit salad, you will need the following ingredients: ½ head curly lettuce leaf (tear it into small pieces), ½ head of red lettuce leaf (torn into small pieces as well), 1-2 avocadoes (slice them beforehand), 1 large grapefruit (remove all the segments from the membranes), 1/3 cup raw walnuts, 1 cup sunflower sprouts and a dash of mint for serving.

Also, you will need some ingredients in order to make the dressing as well. These ingredients are the following: 1 large grapefruit (juiced), 1 navel orange (juiced), 1 large lemon (juiced), 1/3 cup raw cold pressed sunflower oil (you can also use olive oil(, 1 ½ tablespoon agave syrup, ¼ teaspoon honey mustard, a pinch of celtic salt and ¼ teaspoon grated ginger (fresh is preferable).

Start by making the dressing and then combine the different types of vegetables in the ingredients list. Use only 2/3 out of the entire dressing quantity and, if you want to, sprinkle everything with chopped mint and/or with extra walnuts.

Creamy and Green Smoothie

Smoothies are an excellent way to start the morning and they can make for a very good snack as well. Even more than that, they are full of vitamins and healthy nutrients, most of them are fully alkaline and they will satiate your hunger when you do not have the time to cook yourself anything else. Do make sure that you do not add any kind of sugar, that you do not add cream or full fat milk and that you only use fresh ingredients. Furthermore, never make your smoothies much in advance because they will lose their nutrients.

To make this particular creamy and green smoothie, you will need the following ingredients: 1 cucumber, some broccoli stems, 1 stalk celery, some stems of bok choy, a piece of parsnip (3-

4 inches), a small wedge of cabbage and some stems parsley and basil (these ones are optional).

Making this smoothie is the same as with every other smoothie: add the ingredients to your blender and mix them thoroughly until you obtain your smoothie. You can serve as such, you can sprinkle a bit of basil or parsley on top or you can also serve it with ice as well (good especially for those hot summer days).

Crunchy Salad

If you are in the mood for something crunchy and healthy at the same time and if you do not have much time at your disposal to put together something more elaborate, then this salad will be absolutely perfect. Every single member of your family will love it regardless of whether or not they are on the alkaline diet as well!

To make this salad you will need two sets of ingredients. The first one is for the salad proper and the second one is for the dressing. For the salad, you will need the following things: 6 purple stripe beans (chop then finely), 1 cup finely chopped red cabbage, 1 finely diced candy cane, 5 finely chopped radishes, 1 lemon cucumber (dice it beforehand), ½ cup jicama (dice it finely beforehand) and 2 apples (peel them and dice them beforehand).

For the dressing, you will need the following ingredients: ¼ cup olive oil, ½ lemon (juice), 3 drops of stevia, 1 tablespoon finely chopped fresh thyme, 1 tablespoon finely chopped fresh stevia (this is optional) and a pinch of sea salt.

Making the salad itself is very easy: simply chop everything and mix well together. As for the dressing, bring together all the ingredients and then leave the mixture aside so that the flavors combine with each other. Pour as much of this dressing as you want to.

Of course, these are just some of the recipes that can be made with alkaline products. There is an absolutely huge variety out there and as long as you try to keep away from the bad acidic foods and to stick to those that can actually provide your body with something truly beneficial. Allow your creativity to burst and cook things that are healthy, alkaline-friendly and tasty as well!

Conclusion

Changing your lifestyle is not easy, but in most of the cases out there, it will be something you will absolutely have to do no matter what. Changing your diet to one that is more in accordance with the alkaline theory will bring you enormous benefits and it can turn your life upside down (but only for the better).

The best part about the alkaline diet is that it is not a restrictive diet like many out there. You will be allowed to eat almost anything you wish for (except for processed foods, soda and store-bought sweets that contain unrefined sugar). However, at the same time, you will notice changes such as the following ones:

Your skin will look rejuvenated
You will feel rejuvenated yourself as well
Your digestion will be much improved
Your bone structure will grow stronger

You will decrease the chances that you develop certain very commonly encountered diseases and medical conditions (such as arthritis or digestive system-related medical conditions

You will have much more energy

You will decrease the chances you develop cancer

The list of benefits could go on and on. The main point of the alkaline diet is that you really have to balance out your nutrition. Too much acid in your body can lead to the development of many medical conditions (especially according to the latest studies made in the field). At the same time though, you will have to make sure that you do not exclude acidic foods completely from your life (unless you suffer from a very serious disease – case in which you should try to go almost entirely alkaline).

The most important thing to keep in mind throughout the entire lifestyle changing process is that you have to be positive. Start out with a positive attitude and always maintain it no matter how hard things may be. Being optimistic truly helps and it can truly help you stick to your new lifestyle!

Smile, because this diet should not feel like a punishment. On the contrary though, this diet should be something that will teach you just how strong you are. This diet will change your life for the better. This diet is the first step you will have to make towards a truly new life.